# knot body

T0054306

knot body
© 2020 Eli Tareq El Bechelany-Lynch

Published by Metatron Press
Montreal, Quebec
www.metatron.press

Printed in Canada

Second printing

Editor | Tess Liem
Cover art | Lee Lai
Author portrait | Lenore Claire Herrem

Library and Archives Canada Cataloguing in Publication

Title: Knot body / Eli Tareq El Bechelany-Lynch.
Names: Tareq El Bechelany-Lynch, Eli, 1994- author.
Description: Poems.
Identifiers: Canadiana 20200222260 | ISBN 9781988355214 (softcover)
Classification: LCC PS8639.A735 K66 2020 | DDC C811/.6—dc23

We acknowledge the support of the Canada Council for the Arts, which last year
invested $153 million to bring the arts to Canadians throughout the country.

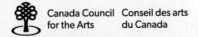

# KNOT BODY

ELI TAREQ EL BECHELANY-LYNCH

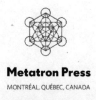

**Metatron Press**

MONTRÉAL, QUÉBEC, CANADA

# knot body

## Portrait Of A Body In Pause

## Portrait Of A Body On Fire

# Portrait Of A Body In Transit

# Self-Prescribed Bed Rest

For my sister Kristeen,
who has always been my biggest supporter

# knot body

"Sometimes to give a person a word to call their suffering is the only treatment for it."

- Anne Boyer, *The Undying*

# Portrait Of A Body In Pause

Dear friends, lovers, and in-betweens,

I anticipate showing up today, fresh and clean, the energy of yesterday and tomorrow running through my pores, and yet—dismissed before the first step out of bed, so who knows how this will go. She tells me to take a bath to soothe my stomach but I hate baths, the hot water burning my skin, the heat making me dissociate. Where did I go? Away, far and out of the bathroom, and maybe down the hall, in your room, or perhaps theirs, or perhaps at the foot of the fridge peaking in, and leaving the light on too long. *Hey*, he yells, *you're wasting energy. Close the damn door!* Or was that yesterday? The days fog and blur, but you tell me it must be Friday if the light is looking this faded. Today, I walked out the door in my biggest coat and sweat all the way down the street, wet between my toes, my socks dewy. At the end of the street, the man walking towards me wouldn't move and as I approached, he said *hey, wait a second, don't I know you?* But I will not be tricked this time by eyes so fakely tender. Lo and behold: a yell, *bitch*, behind my back, and what of this nonsense when it starts snowing and I'm still sweaty. They say just in a day's work, as though we all know the drill and somehow that's it. In the future, we might not need to stop making eye contact with men. In the past, we might not have entered spaces with men. Who are we? I'm not sure, but somehow we are not men. I mean, what of the pain in my legs as I shuffle quickly to the bus, a tension in the backs of my calves that only stops when I slow to a glacial pace. None of this will do, the bus is coming in 3 minutes. Well here we are, hoping January ends soon, because we all know what's coming next.

The days get brighter but somehow I don't. A dilemma, right? I thought I was swayed by the light, moods lifting as the clouds lift, yet this pain is fingers deep. My plants grow white bugs and my fingers grow internal bugs and we all just try our best. Why do I feel so lazy as I waste away in bed? The exercise it takes to jump through this is enough. I roll around a Lindt dark chocolate in my mouth and feel luxurious.

Feel free to visit me as I try to feel better.

xoxox,
Eli

# Portrait Of A Body In Pause

It does not start the way you imagine. The last breath is the first breath, the lungs stretched to their capacity, and yet too little air makes its way through. The breath hitched, strangers looking back to see you walking towards their backs, quick enough for your shins to stiffen, to forget you have a body long enough to make that last sprint and catch the bus before it rushes off.

You sit up straight on the bus seat and avoid the white lady glares, but you're sitting too straight and looking away with your neck in that crooked way, and you feel it shooting signals all the way down your back. Trading one avoidance for another.

The shame takes a backseat. When was the last time you had the luxury of forgetting about your body?

I am desperate for a larger vocabulary to talk about my pain. The difficulty with writing about pain is trying not to use the word pain too many times. I keep hitting command + F to make sure pain makes up less than 10% of my word count.

I start keeping tabs of all the words I use:

1. stinging
2. picky
3. burning
4. stabbing
5. aching
6. scalding
7. pounding
8. radiating
9. waves
10. bolts
11. stretching
12. flashing
13. pins and needles
14. splitting
15. nauseating
16. searing
17. tearing
18. cramping
19. gnawing
20. pulsing
21. sore
22. constant

When I ask my pain if it has any consideration for my poor nerves, it replies. "You mistake me, my dear. I have the utmost respect for your nerves. They've been my constant companion these twenty years."

I read about illness as metaphor, writers in pain worrying about falling into clichés. We can either talk about illness bluntly, in plain words, or address the pain metaphorically, or even, surprisingly, in beautiful ways. Is it too hard to believe in this multiplicity while bent over the toilet, throwing up the ache in your stomach? We retch and retch and the pain doesn't fade; it transforms.

Anne Boyer says: "It was in this brief period that I could hold a visceral memory of having been miserable firmly enough to appreciate almost being sick no more than I experienced something like happiness".

What of the moments between pain and relief? I'm not trying to say we should feel lucky for pain so we can understand happiness through the experience of no pain. But what of feeling joy in these moments because we are enmeshed in the pain anyway? Is happiness always just the feeling of relief?

I once thought my worries about my chronic pain stemmed from the fear that I would no longer be able to do the things I have always done. But my bed, a new site for pain, is also for napping, for reading, for looking at my phone for hours instead of sleeping, for depression, for studying, for fucking, for gay processing, for asking is this a date or is this not a date as my leg gently touches her leg, for injecting T, for watching TV (living rooms often unoccupied), for laughter, for swallowing Venlafaxine XR pills, for language, for the can you pass me your water because I drank all of mine, for the sharing of snacks whenever someone comes over, for can we eat in my bed because my kitchen table hurts my back, for staring blankly at the wall.

The pain hovers above an impossible memory. We excavate the impossible memory, a large dark spot neither of us can see clearly. The impossible memory is vague, obscured, not by disorder, but the dimness of the light in the room, our eyes having a hard time adapting. The examiners, me and you, are confused and inquisitive. We dash in close and peek at the impossible memory, peer over hedges and fences built to keep it safe. But it is impossible, and the root of the impossible is that it is not possible. Excuse my obviousness, but sometimes we cannot see the obvious until it is broken down into smaller pieces. The impossible memory has a rich and heavy interior, but we can't see anything. We sense the richness and the heaviness. You look at me and my adrenal glands are activated. My heart is activated, my lungs are activated, my facial muscles twitch. My GI tract slows down and my executive functions disengage. I ask you how you can see inside of me. What are you? You say, never mind that silly, let's keep looking.

We run back and forth until we're dizzy with sweat and adrenaline, with fatigue and failure.

We pretend it doesn't exist but the impossible memory keeps reminding us it does.

I scream, please tell me, please tell me, please tell me.

It ignores me. This is not how it works.

I worry that in writing this, I am revealing too much.

For some writers, the memoir is a space of control, a way to reveal the facts they want to reveal, to share their stories so others know they are not alone, to share their stories in the hope that they are not alone. I try to learn from other writers, and give small parts of me, dropped into a glaze of fiction, fired twice over until the reality of it all changes colour, a lilac purple into raw clay brown. Charles Baxter says poets don't particularly care about the study of character so I guess he's never met a poet. Tommy Pico would rip him to shreds. Mix around some random details and turn myself into a character, so far away from me that I can convince both you and I that nothing bad has ever happened to me.

# Portrait Of A Body On Fire

Dear friends, lovers, and in-betweens,

I don't know about you but sometimes I forget how to feel joy. ·
Yeah, just that, no big deal. In the waves in Cuba, my friend
and I wonder how to feel at peace, how to feel in the moment,
letting ourselves get hit by the waves, our skin sizzled by the
sun, our limbs coated by the sea salt. My favourite place is the
beach and yet somehow I want to be at home, remembering
the beach. They say they understand and so we sit in silence,
meditating with the waves, hoping we can feel some kind of
spiritual connection, as though we can will it into existence,
but we both know we're full of shit. So we plan our trip to
Lebanon, and think up ways of being as gay as possible in the
country we both love and hate.

Returning to winter, I keep writing about my pain, sitting on
the couch to support my back, never eating soon enough to
avoid the shakes. Writing about pain only brings more pain,
throwing me out of that sweet dissociation I live in every day.
Am I sacrificing my joints to be a poet?

Being present is the most difficult, dissociating such a treat,
our bodies smarter than we think. My body really trying to
keep things productive for me because it knows I'm living in
capitalism. The reminder of a body is not always useful when
trying to live.

I remember my mother's warnings, the ways she expressed
joy when giving. My mother doesn't act resentful but I still
feel the resentment growing in her. My mother has always
shared a room with many, shared her toys with many, shared

her money with many, shared her food with many, shared her heart with many. I close my heart a little bit more, the way my father showed me, but I don't know which method is worse.

I walk on the snow and my pain flares up so much, I can barely breathe. Seems weird since I feel so calm but I've mostly learned not to wonder why right now, because it never really makes sense. Fibro is resting bitch face, and you can't always see what's underneath. I stop and breathe deep. I breathe so deep I can almost taste the pee in yellow snow. In this moment, I wish I was a dog and that somehow pee did something for me. Or maybe I wish I had a pee fetish. Then this might feel ok. Instead, I smell pee and weakly ask you to slow down, wait for me please. We stand around, and you smell pee along with me, though your nose is further away, my head in between my legs. Breathing exercises have never been so disgusting.

Remember to breathe, friends! You never know when it'll be a bonding moment. The winter works in mysterious ways.

xoxox,
Eli

# Several Rages

After Vi Khi Nao's 'The Binchōtan Charcoal & Its Ash'

I am often inspired by attention.

I take several walks a day to remind myself what energy feels like
Inspired by your openness, I go on long tangents

Am I to be left in this bed?

She tells me if you see me more often, something might change
She says, but what of the chokehold you put me in
the disinterest in your fingertips as they slipped from around my throat

She doesn't look me in the eyes

She opens her mouth once again but this time
nothing comes out

Her fate is that of a dream
Sadistic dependence willing it all to end
It's a place in my head

Sometimes a made up diagnosis
feels like the only solution

They are transfixed by the idea of morphing
plucking themself out of their own body
or perhaps mutating into something more malleable

The pain hums
lactic acid in the muscle of their thighs
the heavy limb weighed down on the bed
they fall asleep with a few fingers perched
gently between the last two pages of their book
their freshly cut hair spiked up
by the push of the pillow
and the dampness of the threads

Time is ever-changing when in pain

She let them hold her hand
before leaving for good this time

She seems like a fiction of their imagination
but she is solid
built of bones, muscles, and flesh
like the rest of us

When was the last time they felt restful?

An attempt at bed
ushers in the threat of insomnia

They sighed long enough to encapsulate
the next moment of relief

Several rages make her delusional

What is delusion but a way of reminding us
we are not mentally fit enough
to speak out loud without offending

Offense without defense is poor sport

Is this how contradiction is born?

She only offends those who don't seem to know
That beauty can exist
in several tiny compartments

Her bed is a king
big enough to welcome several guests
or just herself on a restless night

Her God doesn't exist
if They did, she might not have this throbbing headache
this pulse in the bottoms of her feet

She is dissatisfied

The only virus she lets in
is the one that can't compete

Dear friends, lovers, and in-betweens,

If I could look at the inside of my body, I would. I might even show you. Is the rotting pain in my stomach actually visible as it flinches, jerks, pinches, needles? The writhing pain in my back that won't stop twitching, what's that look like from the inside? My joints, are they actually the way I imagine them, lacking enough fluid between them, the bones just clashing against each other, bone damaging bone, two files whittling each other down? I don't really care if you believe me except I need those meds to sleep. Need that prescription to keep being refilled, need to stand in line at the pharmacy with all the other old people. Downloading the Jean Coutu app changed my life! Did you know you can order your pills online? I only found out because of Grace and Frankie.

Frankie standing in a huge line that made her ankles ache, Frankie protesting for the sake of all the other olds. And the pharmacist screaming, you know you can fill out your prescription online, you won't have to wait. Huh.

Three different podcast hosts talk about Rihanna this week, how she sold all the ~ultra-luxury supreme~ copies of her photography books, filled with pictures of her for 90 000 pounds each, only ten in the world. Capitalism feels like a satire of itself. This could be about anyone other than Rihanna. After I write this, Rihanna proceeds to donate over a million dollars' worth of ventilators to hospitals in Barbados, one of the only celebrities to do anything useful during the ongoing Rona crisis, so what do I even know, right? People only judge black people for being rich, as though they should suffer better, while Bezos and Musk are just building up their stink. B. asking people to donate to Amazon workers risking their lives while millions sit in his bank, the monster from Spirited Away needing to relinquish everything inside of them, all their material goods, in a bath of spas, a sauna meant to cure greed.

The day I remember that some people make my yearly income in a day is the day I have two panic attacks walking up the hill, my breath already ragged moving up and down my trachea through my nose and mouth. If I look inside, would I see Pixar characters working hard, pulling at strings to make sure my lungs work, my trachea works, my nose hairs filter debris? Sometimes I think too much about how I'm breathing and then I can't stop focusing, the hill getting bigger and bigger, the top further and further away, every minute a dollar, every second a bomb drops somewhere in the Middle East. My lack of specificity is not about not knowing, it's happening everywhere you look. My mom says *the world always sucks and right now it just really sucks*, as if to say, what were you expecting, and the ways those words sound coming out of her mouth is like an echo of the years spent working and destroying her body. I try to cure myself by lying very still, wasting away in the bed of my fatigue. But I'm always typing, always worrying. If my body can't move quickly, my brain will work overtime to overcompensate.

It so often feels like the demise of capitalism is the cure to all of our problems. Please come up with six ideas to replace capitalism for our next correspondence. It's all riding on you. No pressure!

xoxox,
Eli

# Betsy

Omg, who is she? she's so big and bold
she wears that shoulder so well
a style icon in her own right
they say her name is Betsy
but I can't quite tell what she wants     she lives on the right
a big bowling ball dyke knotting her way into my shoulder
overpopulating my body and the signal wires get crossed
bringing bowling shoes back into fashion
maybe she's excited to meet me, maybe she wants a new friend
but this pain works deeper than a knot
it recirculates in my body     works its way        through
my bloodstream              and muscles
I tell her Betsy
looks like you forgot your bowling ball
right in the space between my neck and shoulders
forgotten slowly        over time
I try to remind her  come back and grab it

Betsy you're hurting

                    me     Betsy forgets

                        she isn't trying to

                            hurt me

lying on the massage table I hear the bubbles of the aquarium,
the hum of your dog buzzing around, in and out of the room
wanting any attention we can give her, before finally, defeated
she settles her butt on a chair, watches me from her perch
we work on Betsy        she's easing her way out
you dig you fingers into my shoulders
into my back, first gently
and then deep and hard
look at the way Betsy gets all nervy and cracky
look at the way it starts to loosen
squeaking like a baby chick
this is the moment I hold back little noises threatening
to escape my mouth because I might sound like I'm enjoying it
too much
the queer fear of being creepy
while someone massages your naked body
the bed sheet tucked into my underwear
every other piece of my body exposed

we can work with them now
my stubborn knots are trying to talk
but it's a language I don't understand
hey Betsy, speak English
I feel like the Franco police in Quebec
soften my voice, relax into the pain
I tell her French or Arabic works too
I kind of know Spanish?
but Betsy and I only know the language of pain
and so we push harder against her
until it becomes too much

I talk to Betsy at night, rub her, remind her about her bowling balls
Betsy and the bowling balls are one, they cannot be separated
she's a hard Taurus eager to please     but stuck
she won't move until she knows where she's going
when I massage her I don't know where to tell her to go
so she stays     smaller  and smaller


                          but still there

Dear friends, lovers, and in-betweens,

I listen to this mix on repeat.

The mix is a consequential and life-changing mix, a meld of all my friends, lovers, and in-betweens, past, present, and possible futures. I wasn't sure if I would have to reveal the contents of this mixtape to reveal its complexity. What if this mixtape was just the thought of the mixtape, at least for you, and the mystery of its contents would keep you guessing for months? Maybe you make a mixtape to emulate my mixtape, attempting to get the right combination of sad and joyful, of smooth and upbeat, the kind of mixtape we could listen to in the car with the windows down or at home, with the sound just loud enough to hear it from the kitchen.

The first song is slow, probably instrumental, or maybe it doesn't have lyrics but you can hear a voice in the background, one made of noises and sighs rather than words, an Arab tonality, the grandiosity of Oum Kalthoum with the popularity of Nancy Ajram. Neither of these women are featured in the song however.

Maybe the second track is unlike any you've heard before. I don't claim to be a music expert so I will spare you an explanation of its sound. All I can say is that it leaves you wanting more, just in time for track number three.

Maybe the mid-mix songs will bring you out of the funk of the slow ones before. You were perhaps starting to fall asleep, thinking this one might be a yawn fest and questioning the integrity of this mix. I watch a video of this queer couple in purple, several shots of them dancing, one in a dress, one in a power suit, both with glitter and purple lipstick, to the words my sugar bae. The mid-song on the mix is not this song.

The next song is perhaps not so upbeat, it is perhaps the glow of a golden hour, the sunlight on your closed eyelids when you can no longer look at a screen. I live in careful proximity to my neighbours on a cul-de-sac where all the old Greek women and the old South-Asian ladies gossip from each other's balconies, an orchestra leading you to the next track.

The mix is dependent on the intended audience. You who are reading this might not be the intended audience, though perhaps you might also be this intended audience. It is unclear to me who is reading and who is not, so we must live under the assumption that you are not the intended audience. We must also live under the assumption that you are.

I might skip describing many of the next tracks because they are not so different from the fifth and the sixth and the seventh. This is called cohesion. The tracks are only different enough to move the narrative forward but not so different that the listener is derailed. No, we must keep the cohesion, the pretense of chaos without the overall effect. But don't get me wrong, this is a no-skip mixtape.

The last song is only for you, the one you who might not even be reading this. Only you will know what the last song sounds like.

Then again, perhaps the last song does not even exist.

You didn't think I'd reveal all my secrets, did you?

xoxox,
Eli

Dear friends, lovers, and in-betweens,

My favourite food is fried chicken. Take a well-cooked piece of fried chicken and watch that juice squirm out, hot in your mouth, burning your tongue. I keep forgetting my probiotics, so the oil from the chicken coats my gut. Apparently, there's something called a fibro diet, one where you eat things that are good for your gut, things that don't cause inflammation. Stay away from junk food. Seems easier said than done. I start eating oatmeal every morning, warm up apples, sprinkle it with cinnamon. But you see, this is where I get caught. All the websites tell me to eat healthier.

Let's not play the blame game, let's not talk about food as healthy or unhealthy, let's not talk as though we know more than we do, let's not talk about diets, let's not talk about the gym, let's not talk about running daily, let's not talk about eating clean, let's not talk about being dirty, let's not talk about the "right kinds of fat", let's not talk about proportions, let's not talk about pear shapes and apple shapes, let's not talk about fat in women and fat in men, let's not talk at all.

xoxox,
Eli

Dear friends, lovers, and in-betweens,

I anticipate the taste of iron, and stop just before I taste it, leaving myself hanging on the scent of it. I don't write about love in poetry because I'm afraid of being a cliché, so I write about sex and become the biggest cliché of all. I tell you, I need space, but boundaries are hard to press down onto, put into place, spread apart. If I tell you I don't want to have sex, will you tell me it's okay? The vampire in me draws you in, but as soon as I have you, I don't know what to do with you. The only way I know desire is to watch you salivate over me, as I smell the blood moving forcefully through your veins. I taste blood tinged with estrogen and wonder when you started transitioning. I don't ask and you tell me when you're ready. Your favourite part of this agreement is that I don't ask too much. I hold in my curiosity, going against my nature to please you. When you start using she pronouns, they slip off my lips effortlessly. There has always been something of the feminine in you waiting to burst out, so no one is surprised, even less so me, because you are as you have always been. *No, what I mean to say is when the sun beats down right across your face, it's a really good way for me to forget the day ahead of me.* Your black hair sways as you walk away, kissing the top of my head. You are moving too far away, it's almost too much.

Please email me from Hong Kong, and tell your mother I say hi.

xoxox,
Eli

# The Siphon

We sat on our balcony, on the top of the mountain, and looked down onto all the little cars moving. Here, there is nature among cars, foliage and roads, a city below us small and ant-like in its distance. It is proximal enough to imagine hearing our cousin screaming at his mother in their crowded apartment.

Closing my eyes, I hope for something to shift. You tell me to keep my eyes closed and imagine a siphon. You say, when people die, imagine them as a grain of sand floating back to the top of the siphon, joining all the souls in grain form, slowly inching closer to the bottom of the siphon, the sand of time actually the accumulation of our lives, and one day, we will become another.

Can you imagine anything more beautiful?

The Beirut mixed media skyline tries to measure up, the combination of tall condos and old buildings restored anachronistically, everything smoother and shinier than it ever could have been.

I left the marble floors behind and realized the weight of the air around me. It got colder, the particles in the air growing dense with water. I shivered in the deepness of my breath and went inside to call my Teta. She didn't answer, no one answered, the house uncharacteristically empty.

Long ago, my Teta was given to a man twice her age. At fifteen she had her first child, a boy birthed in pain, the weight of the birth forgotten when his gender was discovered, a boy on the first try, a legacy to be proud of.

Pain running through her veins, it touched all three children, women or queered, left a hard stone in each of them, a stone passed on. How many centuries have we lived in the pain of war? How many have felt as bad as this? The stone became a bomb, and the bomb became a violation, and that violation was passed on through red blood cells, through DNA, through pain receptors present all over the body. Salvage our souls and throw them back into the hourglass, do we return with our pain? Are the new bodies holding their own ancestral wound? What happens when they mix? Does the reaction burn through the newly created skin?

Dear friends, lovers, and in-betweens,

Exceptionalism is the lie we tell ourselves to keep pushing towards an unachievable goal. You sit at the foot of my bed and watch me from your perch but don't touch me, just give me that look that says, stay right there. You are not frightened, no, more observant. The cool distance of your body contrasts with the heat in my own. Today, I tried on six pairs of pants at the store to no avail. What is the difference even between a size 12 or 14, a size 38 or 40? It's all arbitrary, even though someone tells me if I can fit the length of my forearm in the waist hole, that it should fit, but have they heard about fat? It's not like my arm grows in length when I gain more weight. Half the battle is hoping the weight I gain is in a place deemed appropriate by pant makers. For some reason, they think my ankles are where all my fat should go while my thighs should stay petite. Did you know there's something called a straight size? It's just not a plus size. I'd rather be plus than straight. I'm even too gay for clothing.

The lies we tell ourselves so we can get up in the morning. Sometimes I just sleep over at your house so you can help me get up in the morning. The number of times a loved one has made breakfast for me is innumerable. How do I redistribute the weight of those acts? I start making mental charts of what is given to me and what I owe, the list growing into an intricate spreadsheet, so long and complicated that I can no longer hold it in my brain. I stop myself from writing it all down in Excel because that's just too much. Of course I can't consider marriage when I'm lying face first in bed. The only act of anarchy I can perform from this site is refusing to legally tie my life to another. Would you even want to saddle your sack to this old horse? My polyamorous rad politics make me better than you somehow, right? The you that wants to be legally tied, the you that wants a celebration of love, the you who has chosen just one human to raise kids with. We're all hypocrites when we're not looking hard enough. I buy Perrier, which I hate, for one lover, and my other lover tells me it's genocide owned. If you know me, I'm screaming in the streets daily about Zionism. Am I part of the problem when I've shelled out $1 when it was on sale?

THERE ARE MORE PALESTINIANS OUTSIDE THEIR OWN COUNTRY THAN IN. THERE ARE MORE LEBANESE OUTSIDE THEIR COUNTRY THAN IN. THERE ARE MORE SYRIANS OUTSIDE THEIR COUNTRY THAN IN.

We all come from suffering. Our people separated quickly and efficiently, the way the word efficient sounds good until it's not. I do understand the new difference, the ways our actions can't be changed, the way the Lebanese government and so many of its people have treated Syrians and Palestinians like dirt. And what of our similarities when our differences are solidified through hate? There's this meme of a frog that has the face of the British flag, that asks *Arabs, can you revolt against the Ottomans?* and the Arabs, in the form of a map say, *You promise our independence?* We all know where the meme ends. A people split into pieces, Greater Syria divided by a hard line, the border between Syria and Lebanon. The border between Lebanon and Palestine. Between Jordan. The creation of that ungodly country I must not name.

I don't understand the way your eyes shine when you laugh, sitting on my couch. I don't understand how to tell you this without making me sound creepy. The summer fades into winter in a deadening way, except for the sun, those fall sunsets the deepest pink, the deepest purple, the most orange golden hour, the most painful omission of light. You text me about the fish you caught in your net, fish sliminess in the palm of your frozen hand, the dew sitting on the tops of the blades of grass, just between day and night, the crickets fighting to see who can be the loudest.

The texts I receive always make it into poems so watch out what you say!

xoxox,
Eli

Dear friends, lovers, and in-betweens,

I forgot to take my probiotics for a few days, and my shit got a little runnier. The things going on in my stomach are hard to explain. I'm not a scientist. I just listen to whoever sounds the most convincing. My last roommate told me 50 billion live cultures is where it's at. I take his advice, keep it in my back pocket for years. Every time someone asks about probiotics, I say, 50 billion is where it's at, my tape recorder mouth rewinding for the next time someone asks me. Be confident and you can be convincing.

My aunt takes her health into her own hands. She starts asking her doctor to prescribe her meds for her brain, for the pain, for her stomach, for anything she thinks might not be working. She becomes a pharmacist in her own right. When my sister starts having stomach aches, she tells her, *take this*, and my mom obliges. The skeptic in me rises and a quick Google search shows it's more dangerous than it leads on. I tell my aunt, you are not a pharmacist, and feel shitty while saying it. She crawls into the ball she always goes into when she is being shamed. *You hurt me*, she says, and I can almost see a bruise forming on her arm.

I forget to research the new medicine prescribed to me. I forget to remember its name. I say, I don't care, I can finally sleep. The skeptic in me has been sedated. I'm too exhausted to invest in the research. The sleep deepens, I go into a better state of rest. The grump moves on to bigger and better things. I can once again abuse my body to its limits, because capitalism isn't going to let me stop, especially now that I can stay awake.

Watch me serving coffee again, my legs ready to fall off.

xoxox,
Eli

# I Am Not Looking For A Miracle

Tired boy, fat boy;

wrists and ankles, stiff

the feeling of ache and hardened

and still

in the middle of the poem. Wrists and ankles

at the centre of stiff lines. For the sake of your body

get up! The brain a fog. Think enough

about getting up and you might just think

you're doing it. Picture your body

getting up slowly, first your head moving up

off the pillow, then your shoulders

arms and torso follow

halfway up when you realize

you're still stuck.

The upper half of the body, the lower half of the spirit

a connection broken, rigid in their ancient ways

the rational and irrational brains don't talk.

One shuts off while the other starts pumping adrenaline.

This has happened so often

you don't even feel it.

Your body is always on edge, at rush

the faint reminder of energy in the morning coffee

a faint jog, the time you thought you lost your sister

a shock to the system.

Here then, a story:

you fell down the stairs, rolling faster and faster

among the pictures of Mary and Jesus

the basement dark and yet you could still see

their brightly lit faces, you begged Jesus

begged Mary, on your knees at the foot of the stairs

palms against each other in simulated prayer

please do not appear in front of me

I do not want a miracle, I do not want

your help. They stayed put in the frames

but always you felt them follow you

with their eyes. Here then, another story:

he yelled and yelled so loud

from the top of those stairs

that every muscle in your body contracted

and haven't stopped

contracting since. Here again, a better story:

they held you crying

the first time in years

a breaking, the cracks in the ground

the earthquake of feeling

edging you apart

clawing at your breath

they held on tightly

while you broke apart, over and over

and somehow

they still stayed.

Dear friends, lovers, and in-betweens,

I tell you to come over for two hours and no more because I can no longer sleep properly if someone is lying beside me, cuddling takes up too much energy. I kick the cat out of bed. The sun shines and I wish we were cuddling in the sun, and we text, you in your office, me in my bed. Sometimes I feel so lazy, I can't imagine my body being worth anything other than waste.

I can write exhaustively about my body but if I'm expecting you to watch, am I looking for belief, or for you to see me in pain, up on the stage, twirling as you twist me and turn me in ways that make me ache?

The world is a stage, or so someone whose name I can't remember said, so why not show you my pretty little disorder, and open my body up for all to see. I used to want to be a surgeon, cut and clean, sterilize all the parts and put them back together. Eli Clare says the problem with cure is it depends on a normal, depends on a better used-to-be, and for some of us, nothing used to be different than now, except maybe a little respect we've lost from cowards too fragile to hold us. The normal I want is the normal I get, the kind of sex where I move nothing but my tongue, the kind of sex where I look at you with desire, standing in the bathroom doorframe with only your underwear on, and my eyes tell a story you can easily read.

The responsibility to move from hate to love is a great one, but I'm always up for a challenge.

I'll pencil you in for next Friday, we can process how you felt after I told you I lied that one time about wanting to have sex. Let's say a meeting of 3 to 4 hours?

xoxox,
Eli

Dear friends, lovers, and in-betweens,

This letter is for you as much as it's for me. The moment we look up, the ceiling starts crumbling. Uncanny, isn't it? That the way you look at my face changes my expression, first a mirror of anxiety, then of pain. How did we decide to spend the day together? I move from being a big old grump to a teddy bear with seven days of little blue and pink pills. My snoring gets so loud, you might need to wear ear plugs. The thing about me is, once you know me, you think you know me. But I've moved so much. I need to hold the ground tight or else, it'll feel like floating away. In *The Bisexual*, Leila says, I'm not going to hold your hand, shit or get off the pot, and I had never felt more seen. They had told me, when they first met me, they thought I hated them. She told me, I felt so comfortable around you straight away. I'm not an open door but maybe I can be a mirror. In this poem, I lay around the house waiting for someone to text. Of course no one texts me because I told them not to. IT'S MY ALONE NIGHT, I scream to no one, the words echoing through my room, bouncing off the walls, and hitting me square in the face. I lay in my bed and stretch this way and that way, and the top of my neck to my lower back is a taut wire, and I don't dare move, willing it not to break.

Oops, I almost forgot about you. You to whom I write this letter. Who are you? If not the self-doubt echoing through my thoughts, the internal battle between work harder and please rest. I sharpen my knives to make things easier on myself, but mostly, it's so my guests don't judge me when they come over to my house. My mom would be proud.

Shove everything into the closet, packed and tight.

Is it time for spring cleaning yet?

xoxox,
Eli

Dear friends, lovers, and in-betweens,

The last time I was in Zalka was a trip. My cousin spent day after day monitoring her food intake, watched my sister and I lick our ice cream cones with pleasure, watched us eat without worry. Her diet meant no sugar, no candy, no sweets. It meant no carbs, no bread, no pasta. When we went out to restaurants, she chose the salad with the blandest dressing. I would say I felt bad for her but I used to be her. Have you ever calorie counted? Have you ever stopped eating after six pm? When you tell me you're giving up brown sugar, I have to ignore you until I forget that we're even eating, forget the calories, forget bad food. You try to get me to take the Doritos home so you don't eat them and this is when your eating disorder contends with mine. We resolve to eat them together so we both feel in control. What kind of labour goes into pretending? I dye my hair grey to match my Instagram handle, pretend I have a brand I need to uphold, as though my followers aren't just you and my mother.

When I used to try not to eat, I'd get so faint that I felt like I had lost all the blood inside of me. It seemed unimaginable that this didn't mean something was wrong with me. Another time, I biked up a hill with flat tires that I didn't realize were flat, deep pools of sweat burbling over my shoulder blades and my spine, making their way down to the crack of my ass. I blamed myself for getting out of shape and barely made it home in one piece. Years later, my fibro diagnosis finally made sense, the way I called my fatigue laziness, the way I compared myself to others. You tell me that I'm the person with chronic pain who shows it the least. I don't tell you it's because

I learned how to hide any perceived weakness from a young age. I take it as a compliment even though it shouldn't be. My back starts hurting and I can almost feel it screaming *internalized ableism* as it squeaks and cracks. As it begins to grow louder, I shout over it, pretending I didn't hear it. It goes on like this for many years. Do you see how stubborn I am? I tell my therapist I'm my own worst enemy and she tells me, no, that's his voice inside your head. We come to a stalemate, and it takes me two weeks to agree with her. I come back with my tail between my legs and she laughs. *I don't need to be right; I just want you to feel better.* I almost hug her but remember that is unprofessional. So I just tell her I like her earrings, seems like a good compromise.

Try therapy at least once if you can afford it. It helps me get out of bed to hear my therapist's voice over his.

xoxox,
Eli

Dear friends, lovers, and in-betweens,

Standing in front of a pool of hot water, my body is ready for a dissociation that never comes. What a pleasant surprise! I remember the time my hands overheated so much in the low dish sink at work, all wet and wrinkly, my body feeling elsewhere, the heat rising in me, my feet no longer connected to my body. You tell me, *we must first jump into the hot, then the cold, but we mustn't scream.* We wince going into the cold pool while this older lady toughs it out, starts doing the breaststroke. We breathe deeply to remind ourselves our bodies are not being attacked, but I still jump out of the pool before you, not wanting the cold water to touch my junk.

Bessel van der Kolk is in the hands of every queer on the queerest bus in Montreal. The 80 houses them all, reading about trauma and boasting their somatic knowledge. I ask Bessel what it means that I don't fight or flight, and he tells me *freeze is most effective for you.* I laugh because it's the winter in Montreal, so we are all frozen, but Bessel doesn't get the joke. He is hard to make laugh, so I try harder, telling him that I forgot a memory but it came back so suddenly that it smacked me right back into bed. My knees start hurting when I walk upstairs. My back hurts when I lean in too much. Bessel asks me why I think pain is funny, and I don't have an answer.

Would my life be less fun if I didn't laugh when my wrists start feeling like those of a person with osteoarthritis? I haven't lived long enough for my bones to wear down over time.

Bessel has no humour, but I decide not to ditch him.

I tell Bessel, I'm only 25! You gotta think it's funny that I feel 80.

Bessel thinks it's sad, and this is when I ditch him.

Kolk in Dutch means pond, depth, abyss, chasm, and vortex.

I think Bessel might be too deep for me.

xoxox,
Eli

# The Fatigue

The Fatigue is just fatigue. It
sprays my body like
a numbing agent. Say the
way I sleep might not be
working, say the way I eat
might not be working.
Hope to god the meds
start working. The other day
she said you need firmer
boundaries. Sometimes
this looks like an earlier
bedtime. Fuel your body
with hope that something
might change. Like a bowl of rice
steaming, put it in your mouth
and huff, too quick, too impatient
but if nothing changes, keep
moving. A challenge is only a challenge
once you stop trying. No, I mean
a challenge is always a challenge
when your body doesn't work right
what is right? They only say
the right side of history when
a few decades have passed. Someday
we will look back and see
much of the same. Say thank you
for your friends and the family that stay
in touch. Was it challenging? Everything is
changing. The fatigue is just fatigue
until it's not.

Dear friends, lovers, and in-betweens,

We all have our boring vices. Mine just so happens to be a good binge watch. And maybe I set up candles on the bedside table to make myself feel nice, the Netflix queue prepared for Self-Care™. The winter season shuts everything down, opens up old wounds, and we bear it all in silence. Under bedspreads and cups of tea, I watch doctors on Grey's Anatomy try to figure out complicated diagnoses while my own pain remains undiagnosed. Dr. Yang spends a six-episode arc trying to figure out how three previously healthy kids all develop cardiomyopathy. I daydream, pretend Christina spends months trying to figure out my pain. Who wouldn't want that kind of attention? I won't lie, I also daydream about her as a dyke, her boss energy feeding the dream.

But I don't have my very own doctor, filled with empathy, gossiping with her friends as I lie still in an MRI machine, wondering if my brain might be where they find it. We all have our fantasies. Some think about sex, others a diagnosis so they can scream in their doctor's face, say, HA, I told you something was wrong. I was right. We are not all made equal. Sometimes we are made Virgos with a knack for keeping a grudge.

Don't worry darlings, I promise to try harder to loosen up, do a few yoga poses to ease the pain. But every doctor I see tells me to lose weight, as though a few extra pounds is the source of all this. What does a few even mean? The words weigh on me, ways of seeming not like those other fat people. But fatphobia is the vice we all hold on to, pretend health is our utmost concern, not the hottest men alive on the front pages of magazines with their lean muscles and their six packs. Aren't they just stomach rolls that hurt more when you punch them? Beats me what we're all trying to do. Imagine spending your whole life worrying about your weight. I still can't see a scale without cringing. When the student doctor says, you don't want to weigh yourself, do you, during my routine checkup, it's the first time I'm given a choice.

Bet you thought I was in bed again. Psych, I've finally made it to the studio, writing to you from my uncomfortable desk chair.

xoxox,
Eli

Dear friends, lovers, and in-betweens,

I often feel more in pain while writing. I don't quite have the right setup for my computer and my shoulders and neck tend to ache more. I often push myself to keep writing and get absorbed, forgetting to eat. Often there is someone in my studio eating, passing me half a clementine, or telling me to stretch and I feel grateful for care in those small ways. Is this why we nag those closest to us? I write and write until my brain folds, and the fog feels more like numbness than pain, more faded than my brain can stand. You ask me a question but I'm not there. You say, *Eli, let's go get some tacos at Frida*, but I don't register until you're right beside me. *Hey, Eli.*

*Hey Eli*, as we walk through the people to get to our chairs at the reading. There are no chairs left so we sit on the floor, your feet aching, my back aching. So few queers I've met are truly 'abled'.

Isn't that a bonus for the somatics of pain?

xoxox,
Eli

Dear friends, lovers, and in-betweens,

I dress as best I can each morning, aesthetics integral. What would happen if I looked or felt ugly? Trans people are never allowed this luxury. A transition is always a makeover but more expensive. Can't straighten our hair like Mia Thermopolis and hit those beauty standard nails on the head. Try twice as hard if you're disabled. My own standards have always been plenty. Inhaled them from the world and they sit proudly in my belly. You told me fat was bad and it's just waiting to be proven wrong. Do I have to look good while lying down, drool leaking down my face, my hair spiking up from going to bed with wet hair, my t-shirt torn and bloody from my fourth nose bleed of the week!

If you're sick of hearing about my bed, come check it out, it's pretty comfy. My mom helped me buy it 7 years ago and it's still going strong. My subletter four years ago made a hole in the bottom so I can no longer flip it for maximum use. I never asked him what he did. Don't ask questions you don't want the answers to.

Like I said, catch me in my bed.

xoxox,
Eli

Dear friends, lovers, and in-betweens,

*The resemblance is uncanny. Are you two related? It's just some-thing in your dark eyes, the way you both stare.* Endlessly, you're asked about your relationship, what you are to each other and what you aren't. Shame to be an in-between. The ways you can't quite articulate your proximity, your distance, the bits that feel just right. You anticipate more questions but they never come, because there is something so alienating about the two of you together. People don't like what they can't understand. In the '80s, my mother travelled far away from home, and because she did well in English classes, she felt ready for this new adventure. But a new world is never like an old world, every intonation different, every gesture of approval or disapproval switched. The pain showed up in her arm, years later, and she didn't quite understand the connection, but I told her it was there.

Or is she on to something? Maybe nothing makes sense, I'm trying to fabricate meaning from nothing. I try to piece together pain and cause, as though it could ever lead me to cure. When I feel less pain, it is always a relief. When I feel less depressed, I could almost bounce off the wall. It is midnight but I still want to hang out. I text a few people, tell them it's not a booty call, I promise. We head out, climb Mount Royal, and sit around talking until the sun rises. I take several drops of CBD and lean deep into the green grass, oh wait, had I said it was winter? Okay, wait, actually, we are in my bed again, and I take several drops of CBD, and lean in deep into my cushion-topped bed. You smoke a bit outside my room because I hate the smell of it, and we joke about nothing. When you're ready to sleep and we turn off the lights, I keep talking, and you laugh, tell me to shut up. But of course you're on board and we laugh until sunrise, getting out of bed to watch it, each with a blanket over us like little body tents.

*As the sun rose up, you started speaking a language foreign to both of us. Moving it around in your mouth gently at first, then quickly, you surprised me with the agility of your speech. What you said, I couldn't remember, but your mouth moved in such a pleasing way. Your affect blurred with this new language, some new creation of your mouth, the spit moving around, the click of your tongue, your tongue against your teeth. I sat there and you talked about nothing, and we stayed that way for hours.* This time is almost like that but not quite. The sense you make is abundant. I realize I know you better with every sunrise.

The irony is that this has never happened, drifting between awake and a dream, but a poem might will it into existence. I'll paint a beautiful scene, watch it gleam and shine, present the perfect sentence and everything might be alright. It's like trying to get out of bed. If I visualize it enough, one day it will happen.

I am getting out of bed.

I am getting out of bed.

I am getting out of bed.

I pick my head up.

I am getting out of bed.

I am getting out of bed.

I am getting out of bed.

I elevate my torso.

I am getting out of bed.

I am getting out of bed.

I am getting out of bed.

I swivel my legs off the bed.

I am getting out of bed.

I am getting out of bed.

I am getting out of bed.

I am sitting up straight.

I am getting out of bed.

I am getting out of bed.

I am getting out of bed.

I get up.

xoxox,
Eli

# Portrait Of A Body In Transit

# holding the b0dy

those who cannot forget the past are destined to remix it. - Evie Shockley, *The New Black*

his is the way I wash my body

vash my body     wash my body

        this is the way I wash my body

       of everything  but tender thots

investigating       does this feel good    does this feel good    does this?

       the way i'm always on stage

          you're all looking at my b0dy

       out back and off the stage    laid open

and O the little lilacs coming out       striking but still feeling that lack?

    how often I'm left ajar       open and seamless    an invitation

fraying at the joints    like those pants bulging    growing

       my dad screams THUNDER THIGHS  across the room

          (my dad weighs less than me)

      holding my b0dy      locked in

patch those thighs from chub rub

but that chub will keep on rubbing

and those pants will keep on        breaking

and you will never be held tightly for long

where did I go wrong?

this is the way I wash my body

wash my body wash my body

this is the way I wash my body

of starving on a diet

how tragic to be        such a slender thread of a person

how tragic to give up carbs

(when bread tastes so good)

remember:        fat = good        fat = good        fat = good        fat = GOD

don't try that diet shit on me        don't try that shame shit on me

get out of my house!        yeah I said it

how dare I be so bold

THUNDER THIGHS          yeah I said it

how dare I be so bold

a b0dy a b0dy a b0dy

do you believe in animosity?

do you believe in heaven?

for the next generation?

fat     thickened    laid out          like a prize to be won

this is the way I wash my body     wash my body     wash my body

this is the way I wash my body

of  knots          knots          NOT

I am a knot        of what you think

how tragic to be so cemented in sex          or a gender sexed

the b0dy so bold and free

starting to fray along the seams  edges, a ridge of empathy

but tell me really, is anyone cis these days?

this is the way I sometimes feel ~~like a girl~~ when you touch me

73

but only when you touch me

but I don't tell you

& I don't show you my b0dy

but isn't that the truth and isn't that a mess

and you saying a woman....        uhhhh ladies

won't get me down the way you want it to

*what not a woman?*     yes that's the truth

*and what not a man?*     o yeah that's true too

*like is that even real?*     guess i'm the proof

the truth                just part of the equation

this is the way I wash my body

wash my body    wash my body

this is the way I wash my body

of everyday knots

pulling pieces apart        to distance fem(me) from me

them them them them them them them

but still pretty       this is the way I hold it close        femme and me

        leaking out of my body                 (just for me)

this is the way I wash my body

        wash my body    wash my body

                this is the way I wash my body          of thickening knots

she asks you does it hurt        your voice        cracking and changing

                constantly on the move        up and down your throat

your vocal chords changing            growing

                twenty times their size          the grinch's heart

you are thickening                        lengthening

                        the larynx testosterone heavy

                        yeah  baby

we like 'em thick, yeah, we said it

        yeah baby                & a rip rip rip of my chest

                a deep gash red                left to heal

        pieces of me plucked out

do i need to spell it out

this body transmorphing

fat lumps of chest

where do they go?

piece of me lying dead

in an emesis basin

kidney shaped and sterile          served on a platter

can we eat you like the placenta?

is this how I give life?

O you it's like i never knew you

left in a plastic bin          marked hazardous

waste of space

but i think i might have known you

why do you look so familiar

damn, did we go to high school together?

# Self-Prescribed Bed Rest

## Self-Prescribed Bed Rest

If fibro is a woman's disorder, and someone who is not a woman has fibro, is fibro still a woman's disorder? Or am I just a woman in disguise?

Spoiler alert: that's just transphobia.

I tried starting this essay wanting to talk about the difference between diagnosis for cis people versus trans people, but then thought, what about Black people's experiences with misdiagnosis? What about Indigenous people's experiences? What about Arabs or South Asians or East Asians or Latinx or anyone else that falls under the large POC umbrella? I recently read about Malone Mukwende, a second year medical student at St. George's University in London, who created a clinical handbook which shows how medical conditions present differently on black and brown skin. For anyone who is light skin, this has never seemed like an issue, but for anyone with skin much darker than the white skin presented in medical books, this could be a matter of life and death. The medical system is failing so many of us, and diagnosis fails when those doing the diagnosing only know the assumed normal, cis, white, thin, able-bodied, neurotypical, and male.

When specifically talking about trans people and fibromyalgia, the presumption that fibromyalgia is a woman's disorder banks on the "fact" that women have lower levels of testosterone than men. This assumption doesn't even encompass the experience of all cis women, let alone anyone else. If we've only just started understanding the way testosterone and estrogen function in different bodies, how am I supposed to believe that there's even enough knowledge to imply that higher levels of testosterone serve as pain suppressants?

When I ask myself why trans people are never mentioned when we talk about chronic pain (everyone talks about women's chronic pain but no one ever includes trans women in their definition of women because transphobia), the answer seems obvious, a kind of laziness, an unwillingness to move out of their comfort zone, a frequent disregard of what life might look like for someone else, what the reality of the world might be if we exploded gender to include more people, to look at the experiences of marginalized people, to understand that diagnosis is bullshit when it frames the conversation around two cisgender genders, around white people's bodies, around an abled body, or a thin one.

Doctors use biology that they don't fully understand to create frameworks and rules for diagnosis that leave so many people undiagnosed, regarded as crazy, making it up, not easily categorized and therefore unimportant, or a burden. I don't necessarily see diagnosis as the ultimate end goal but rather as harm reduction. How can I rag on diagnosis when it allowed me to start taking pills used to treat fibro? When my sleep improved so much overnight that my depression lifted more than it had in years?

Diagnosis is important. Important because it enables so many of us to find ways to cope and live through this capitalist world. The thing about including and thinking about trans people, BIPOC, disabled people, fat people, neuroatypical people, and anyone else deemed non-normative, when it comes to all aspects of life, especially in the medical system, is that it helps us stay alive.

& we are not just looking to be seen on tv, we are looking for our meds to be available and covered & we are looking to be believed & we are looking for trans women of colour, for black trans women, to be uplifted to the front, we want safety and love & we want access to meds, to mental health support, access to transition in whatever form it takes.

It is time for so many trans folks to stop dying in such large numbers.

Okay, so at one point, Plato and Aristotle, these two old bearded men, thought of mimesis as the imitation of nature, including human beings, through representation. Mimesis might look like anything put on stage, on the page, in the present day. Plato also thought that poets were mad and didn't speak the truth so maybe he was a bit unreliable. Maybe he thought we were all acting, pretending, a semblance of what could be, but isn't. Aristotle though, he thought mimesis was perfect art. What does perfection mean? And does it even exist?

Dionysian imitatio tells us that imitation is but the reformulation of a previous work to rework it, to enrich it, to improve it, to make it better. We browse the current "source text", cis white men, but always, we exit the conversation looking better. If you tell me what to sound like, I'll make it better. If you tell me what to look like, I'll make it better.

& in my family, they all used to tell us the story of the lady of lebanon, up on harissa, prayed to by both muslims and christians, their conviction melding into one story & harissa, she watches us from her shrine, on the way up to the mountains, they say she cried one day, tears leaking down her face, a miracle & they say, she looked upon the limbs of a child in a wheelchair & "healed" them, he could walk, he could run, the happiest boy, the tears of harissa, the top of the mountain, the telepherique we never rode for fear of falling down & I've always wondered how she "cured" them, those sick kids, those kids in wheelchairs when her perch was so inaccessible, circling up and around the statue, stairs I used to run up as a kid, making me huff and puff & the roads in lebanon have sidewalks that turn into streets & the roads in lebanon have two lanes that turn into one, though two cars still have to meet, you always have to honk if you can't see who's coming, the lebanese drivers slowing their usual speed in the dust of the rocky road

but what about me, or those of us with invisible disabilities, where is our "cure"?

how would anyone know we got cured if they can't see our pain?

When people are constantly looking to god for answers, an entity no one can see, why can we not look to our bodies for signs of pain, and believe in a disorder we cannot see inside a microscope or on test results? Has seeing always been believing?

My little sister used to tell me about this green man made out of boogers who would come to her school when we lived in lebanon. The building was an apartment complex converted into a school, with a second-story parking lot converted into a playground where we'd have gym class. She'd tell me stories in which she arrived at school to find the playground converted into an amusement park, rides everywhere—ferris wheel and a small roller coaster, mirroring dream park, the theme park we'd go to in zouk mosbeh. The booger man would come and chase people around the rides, ruining everyone's fun. My mind was her canvas and she was an excellent painter, crafting images so visceral I didn't realize they were her dreams. The more she told me about her adventures with the booger man, the more I believed. Those memories of the booger man faded and only came back to me years later. Four years older than her, how had I believed her so easily? Was the image just so clear that I couldn't help but pull it into our reality? Can we say it wasn't real if it was real for the two of us?

Fibromyalgia often feels like a fabrication: we try to paint pictures of our pain, we excavate metaphors and obscure concepts to describe what we experience—the pin pricks, the stabbing jolts, or we gesticulate with our hands, mirroring the movements of jellyfish through the water, a pain going in and out.

I tend to compare myself to others. This is often a losing battle. But can you tell a Virgo that and have them listen to you? Most of the time, no.

Last year, I spent the worse half of the year reading sappy quotes about grief, trying to feel better in some way by relating to others. The problem with these quotes is that they're often too general. The speedy retreat from my feelings I wanted wasn't going to come that easily. That's why whole books are written, or intricate poems. Still, I fell on several Anne Frank quotes. She said, "I don't think of all the misery, but of all the beauty that remains". How am I supposed to ever feel bad when Anne Frank still sees beauty in the world?

I also spent the last year riding a broken bike. Instead of wondering if the bike had issues, I looked to my body and saw wrong, saw fat, saw inability. Instead of wondering how I went from being an excellent cyclist to one who could barely bike five minutes without tiring, I had just assumed it was me, I was wrong, I was lazy. When I finally told my friend who bikes all the time, she hopped on it and screamed from the end of the street, "how is your bike so sluggish?"

I walk around Parc Ex and the sun touches the buildings quietly with its evening softness, my ankles throbbing from the uneven snowy sidewalks. This particular street hasn't been plowed properly yet. Most of the time I don't blame the streets but my weak ankles. If the man in front of me can walk seemingly okay, why can't I?

I revisit the Anne Frank quote often, wondering what she had that I didn't. How did she figure it out?

We compare our pain to that of others, often to our own detriment.

Don't get me wrong. There is also power in making comparisons. My favourite essays in high school used to be compare and contrast essays. Put two works of fiction beside each other, and see how they play off each other's strengths, each other's weaknesses.

But looking at our pain, we will never be able to weigh ourselves against others at a 1:1 ratio.

If Anne Frank can see beauty in the world, maybe it's more about learning a little something from her about perspective than comparing my pain to hers.

Talking to friends with fibro, they all explain how well they've studied the script, how often they've looked online to find out the common symptoms of fibro even if they don't have them, to try and emulate the perfect patient. When I walked into my doctor's office, I racked my brain for the web md list I read the previous week. And with the dutifulness of a good memory and Virgo precision, I told him exactly how each symptom developed in me. If I sit in a car for too long without moving my legs, I lose feeling in them, they become stiff and painful. My hands and feet feel as though they are riddled with arthritis. He nods his head with every new symptom, ticking off a checklist in his own head.

The science of medicine is often just memorization.

& in the movie, forrest gump is fitted with leg braces, correcting his back, crooked like a question mark, crooked as a politician & the bullies coming for him because he looks different, not normal, wrong, they're screaming in his face, pushing him down, a little boy confused, hurt, nothing to do but let it happen until jenny screams behind him, "run forrest run," the words mimicked on middle school playgrounds, shouted out of buses as the guy down the street struggles to make his way to the stop, the bus pulling away, the erasure of any kind of disability, forrest's fear makes him stronger, his leg braces crumbling as his run becomes faster, so fast that's he's magically healed, the swelling music in the background alerting us to this surprising miracle, running for the rest of the movie, and by the grace of god, this boy is cured.

like kanye of the old days said, "only jesus can save us".

Cure only allows us to see the world as one dimensional. If doctors are looking for a one-track pill to make us all feel better, of course they will try to lump us all into one person, one biology, one being that can spend money for the chance at no pain. People say fibromyalgia is understudied because it is a woman's disorder, and this world of patriarchy doesn't care about women, but what if it is more complex? What if the complexity of fibromyalgia, its roots in trauma and biology, its reliance on multi-approaches to be better understood, is another factor for its lack of study? When the science of medicine is so obsessed with singular tracks, with singular cures, why would any scientist or medical professional care about a disorder that falls so far outside what and how they are trained to understand?

When I research trans people and fibromyalgia, or trans people and chronic pain, no matter how many times I look, the answers are few and far between, the google search coming up empty. I check each day, hoping for different answers, new studies, hoping today is the day new research comes out to corroborate my own theories, but it never does.

& we are reduced to our hormones, the gender assigned at birth, the female or male of it all & i'm not talking about forgetting biology but the cis-centric story of it all is that women have pain & men don't, the cis-centric of it all is that women are weak & men are not, the cis-centric of it is old stories we tell ourselves over & over, first through religion & then through science, the new immovable frontier

Am I a reliable source if the ache of my body tells me a story truer than any I've read?

& we are animals yes & we are mimetic & we are hiding in plain sight, the eastern whip-poor-will, or engoulevent bois-pourri, french for rotten wood, disregarded junk in the pile of dirt on the ground, disguised as lesser than, the little whip-poor-will finding safety in its invisibility

Now let me tell you a story of biology, one backed up by science, maybe this way you'll believe me.

So often, chronic pain is understood as primarily experienced by women. When the research mentions women, we can read between the lines enough to know they are talking about cis women, or afab people. While this can be applied to most diseases and disorders that are known to affect women primarily, I'll limit myself to touching the subject of pain, the thing that occupies my own daily life, as someone who is not a woman.

There are many theories about fibromyalgia, often interconnected, often defined as a neurological disorder. This is where the idea that fibro is "all in your head" have come from.

Many consider chronic pain, particularly fibromyalgia, a consequence of repeated trauma. When you've experienced repeated trauma, something like being physically or verbally abused over a long period of time, the part of your brain doctors colloquially call the logical part shuts down, and your reptilian brain (or instinctual brain) starts firing off, increasing the dopamine produced by your body. When the trauma continues over a long period of time, your body's instincts and survival tactics change, often from fight or flight to freeze. In these moments when your dad is yelling at you from the top of the stairs, your body tenses up, gets ready for the thing you are expecting. While you may look calm, your body is firing off signals, telling itself to do the things you'll need to survive. Since you are frozen, none of the energy your body has created is used through activities like running away or fighting. It just sits inside of you, a balloon filled with too much air, ready to explode.

But you don't explode, you're tied up just before you inhale too much air, and that air hums in your body, not released through your ears, not through your nose. When your body becomes so used to protecting itself in this way, it becomes hyper-vigilant. When it becomes hyper-vigilant, anything deemed a threat sends it into a state of protection. Sometimes, this might take the form of a loud car alarm shaking you to your core, your heart speeding up, your muscles tensing up. Often when that tension is released, one might feel extreme moments of pain.

Our understanding of fibro might also be explained by looking into the theory surrounding the fascia, a sheet of connective tissue beneath your skin, that separates your muscles from your other internal organs, that keeps everything held tightly, holding so many parts at once. Some people think that the fascia of people with fibro is inflamed, and with that inflammation, the feeling of full body pain.

The other theory is that a body experiencing fibromyalgia will send pain signals to different parts of your body that are not actually in pain, as there are imbalances in your neurotransmitters' regulation. The chemicals which send signals from the brain to the rest of the body appear to be disrupted in fibromyalgia sufferers. Sometimes, you are just in bed watching High Maintenance when your body tenses up, or your leg feels like it's filled with cement, or the pin pricks return to your arms, and won't leave. The Guy character was just biking down the street, his one-eyed dog in his backpack. There doesn't seem to be an explanation for this.

My own theory is, why not a bit of all of it? Either way, it becomes hard for me to understand why this might be something that only affects women.

One doctor says, "there's a notion among physicians that fibromyalgia is only a female problem, so it's not a diagnosis that's often considered in male patients, and male sufferers are often overlooked." Many experts believe that there are probably many more incidences of men with fibro than the numbers indicate. "Additionally, men tend to see doctors less often than women, especially for generalized pain complaints, many men believe that going to a doctor for vague, hurt-all-over pain is being a little bit of a wimp," notes another doctor. Consequently, the number of men who have fibro is low, but if no one actually talks about their pain, how are we supposed to know it exists? Is staying invisible or ignoring the problem another type of "cure"?

What if we actually looked at men's pain, or that of those forced to enact masculinity from a young age, or those choosing to enact masculinity as protection, instead of hiding it? What if we noticed the ways dissociating from so many parts of themselves does not manifest as a chronic pain, signals firing off in the body, but instead as a hidden pain, trauma that articulates itself as violence, as repression, as bullying, as anger, as a sadness so deep it's not allowed to be shown? As an anger we must not excuse.

Would returning to our bodies, no matter our gender, allow us a deeper understanding of what's going on? Will we see the effects of centuries of white supremacy, colonialism, genocide, shame, fatphobia, classism, and other social barriers and violences on our bodies?

CAConrad says, "few things tire me more/than imagining reincarnation/ a child struggling all over again to not/favor war/ not surrender/to greed".

Few things tire me more than trying to ignore all this pain.

I struggle with writing about these intertwining concepts, struggle with finding a way that feels right, that feels just. I do not want, with my words, to hurt others in my community who are not exactly like me. I know how to write about the experiences of being trans and non-binary, living a life of no gender and all gender, living a life of pain and profound friendship and love. I know how to write my Arab diaspora feelings, and to write about light skin privilege and white-passing. I know how to write my own experiences of racism and fatphobia. But I want to write about trans people and pain, and I want to write it well, in all of its complexities. The experience of trans people with chronic pain, fatigue, and fibromyalgia is vast and varied.

I want to honour the experiences of all the women, especially the trans women, who experience fibro and are not believed. I want to honour the experiences of all the non-binary people in my life whose experiences of fibro does not always equate with womanhood. I want to honour the men in my life who might be too afraid to talk about their pain, because they are taught not to. I want to honour the experiences of those traumatized and living with pain, those who link those two experiences and those who don't. I want to honour the friends getting massages or acupuncture, seeing osteopaths, changing their diets, exercising or not exercising, staying in bed, or pushing their bodies to the limit and regretting it. I want to honour people who have chronic pain but don't know it, disassociating so hard from their bodies that they aren't really sure what's going on beyond their thoughts, beyond their output into the world, beyond being useful to others and capitalism. I want to honour those searching for cure because the pain is unendurable and those who hate the word cure, just wanting a slight relief from pain, who want just a little less pain tomorrow. I want to honour those people who have to work, have to labour, have to feed their kids, have to work ten-hour days, come home in pain to sleep, and wake up in pain and fatigue, starting it all over again. I want to honour those, like me, forced to slow down by the occurrence of chronic pain, by the occurrence of fatigue, by the reminder of a body not made to survive through capitalism. I want to honour all those surviving in the best ways they can. I want to honour all those challenging the ways we are told to live. I want to tell you all, I believe you.

Is diagnosis is necessary when we already have words for our pain, when we can tell what we need because our ankles feel inflamed, our head hurts, our stomachs are turning into knots. Is cure necessary if we know how to soothe ourselves through our pain?

Leah Lakshmi Piepzna-Samarasinha half-jokingly refers to people as those who are disabled, and those who are yet to discover they are disabled. Is dissociation the cause of this yet-to-discover?

Are more of us in pain or ill than we think?

& the birds of imitation, pretending to be the thing that they are not, a luminary song assembled from all the notes they hear, the lyre bird with all its beautiful foliage, taking its name from the male's tail, the female left high and dry though her own abilities shine just as bright, taking on the song of other birds, singing for half of daylight hours, never wholly themselves, but never wholly someone else, letting the voices of others move through them, channeling their powers for survival, but shy, only detected through the beauty of their uniquely blended song as they hide.

In *Brilliant Imperfection: Grappling With Cure*, Eli Clare quotes Susan Wendell who says, "Some unhealthy disabled people... experience physical or psychological burdens that no amount of social justice can eliminate. Therefore, some very much want to have their bodies cured, not as a substitute for curing ableism, but in addition to it."

& we are not the cure, or the shapes we take to survive. we move in packs, visually diverse yet connected at our cores, pieces of truth emerging in group, through laughter, through our own songs intermeshed, through our battle cries, creating the loveliest blend of sound.

Dear friends, lovers, and in-betweens,

I began the day reading bits and pieces from Renee Gladman's *Calamities*. You told me you read bits and pieces to past and present lovers so I stubbornly told you not to read it to me. My childish need to be unique stood before me but I pushed it away. I began my voyage with my eyes closed until I had to open them to read. The day has passed and it is always 3pm before I know it and I haven't even read a sentence. My day only begins with the beginning of Renee's day and the woman-loving-woman energy she infuses into the text. I try to read between the lines but Renee is more complex than most. We dedicate our days in bed to building a new friendship she does not know about. This friendship grows in me, and her meaning less obscure, builds new bridges between my own understanding and hers.

The next morning, I wake, having dreamed of falling in love with an anonymous white man. I only remember the colour of his hair and how much taller than me he was but the feeling I am left with coats my body and I can't shower enough to wash it off. We wake up together and I tell you about the man. You tell me that you will give me time with my dream man while I pick the crust out of one of your eyes and your morning chuckle is sleepy.

We wake and we sleep and sometimes nothing changes. The books beside my bedside table start piling up. I lug my books out of my room to convince myself that they are new. My friend tells me she visits her hallway bookshelf like a bookstore. Missing the bookstore clerks, she perches Facetime-me on the edge of the bookshelf and I tell her, that will be $19.95. But my discount! she demands. Oh yes, I say, that will be $16.95 for you, pardon my mistake.

The insecurity I feel grows until it pops like a pimple, the white head squirting out, half solid, half liquid. I tell you about it and you tell me from 6 feet away, why didn't you just tell me? I tell you I wanted to work it out on my own and you tell me you always want to hear my gossip. We settle for a pretend hug and dismiss the whole thing as fake.

I begin the next day with a meditation, visualize my feet leaving my bed. I imagine a sun salutation, imagine my arms moving in slow circles. I fixate on one point and try to clear my mind. Every time my mind wanders, I wrench it back to the black circle, the circle of nothing. Renee sometimes returns to tell me to relax, but her voice is not nothing and so I shoo it away till later.

It is midnight when I pick up Renee again. She is lighter than before as we've reached page 56. "I began the day wanting to fold the previous essay into this new one because I had learned just after writing it that it was possible to make beautiful, complex structures with paper and you did not need to be an architect to do this." Replace essay with letters. This correspondence has gotten so long that I can't seem to find enough paper. The shops are closed so I make do with the backs of old school forms. Shhh, Renee is trying to sleep.

xoxox,
Eli

Dear friends, lovers, and in-betweens,

Please know that when I am in bed, I am thinking of you. Not in a sexy way, unless that's what we've decided. So sometimes in a sexy way, but mostly in a missing way. I always miss you, no matter how close or far you are. Sometimes I forget to miss you if you've been away too long, and that is my biggest sadness. I think I look at my phone too much but mostly it's to remember you. Send me a text telling me you're on the metro, or taking a shit, or need me to text you out of a panic attack. Send me beautiful selfies of your face, or your desk, or the office dog. When we are far, we can be close if I just think about you enough.

Sometimes my hands turn into claws and the ache stops me from texting. Know then that I still love you. Maybe call me? Maybe wait a little longer? Sometimes I will text you through the pain and I promise that is sacrificial love. I'm not saying it's right. But is love right or wrong?

If you are my mom, stop reading now. If you are my friend, do as you please. The bed is my favourite site for pain. For pleasure. For both. When I'm always in pain, it might be a surprise that I want someone to fuck me so hard it aches? The ways I control my pain are the most delicious.

I stack books by my bed to remember faraway friends. It's not an original thought, but I've always looked at books for salvation, a departure from my body to another in movement, in love, in action, in difference, in change.

Solidarity from my bed to yours. Or your couch, or your wheelchair, or your sitting on the metro while old people glare at you to get out of the accessible seat despite your legs being filled with cement from the inside. Maybe one day we'll know how to love each other in all our dignity.

xoxox,
Eli

# Work Cited

Quoted line on p.20 by Anne Boyer is from *Garments Against Women*.

Quoted line on p.55 by Desiree Akhavan appear in the short TV series *The Bisexual*.

Quoted song lyrics on p.41 are from TASHA's "Snacks".

Quotes line on p.93 are from CA Conrad's *While Standing In Line for Death*.

Quoted lines on p.96 are from Eli Clare's *Brilliant Imperfection: Grappling with Cure*.

Quoted lines on p.99 are from Renee Gladman's *Calamities*.

Quoted lines on p.93 appear in "The Role of Gender in Fibromyalgia: Men and women experience fibromyalgia symptoms differently—here's why." by Jan Sheehan. The first quote is by Patrick Wood, M.D., a fibromyalgia researcher and chief medical advisor for the National Fibromyalgia Association. The second quote is by Tarvez Tucker, M.D., a fibromyalgia expert and associate professor of neurology at the University of Kentucky in Lexington.

Quoted lines on p.15 are from Jane Austen's *Pride and Prejudice*, a line spoken to Mrs. Bennet by Mr. Bennet at the beginning of the book.

The book is indebted to the work of so many authors, Tommy Pico's *Feed*, Leah Lakshmi Piepzna-Samarasinha's *Care Work: Dreaming Disability Justice*, the work of Mia Mingus, Bessel Van der Kolk's *The Body Keeps The Score*, and Johanna Hedva's "Sick Woman Theory".

The poem "The Fatigue" has previously been published in *Room Magazine* issue 43.2.

The poem "The Syphon" has previously been published in *Cheups Magazine*'s first issue.

Most of the book was written in the 3 Tables studio in St. Henri, a space founded and run by Wai-Yant Li, one of my dearest friends, or written from my cozy bed in Parc Ex. Both of these spaces are on the traditional territory of the Kanien'kehá:ka people. The Kanien'kehá:ka are the keepers of the Eastern Door of the Haudenosaunee Confederacy. The island we call Montreal, called Tiotia:ke in the language of the Kanien'kehá:ka, has historically been a meeting place for other Indigenous nations, including the Algonquin peoples. Any time I read, write, live, rest, travel, deal with difficulty, or experience joy, it is with renewed commitment to support the sovereignty of Indigenous people on Turtle Island, and elsewhere. As a mixed white POC, I am not exempt from the legacy of colonialism. I am in solidarity with other marginalized people and commit to using my voice to speak out against what is wrong and to create change.

# Acknowledgements

Dear friends, lovers, and in-betweens, (+family),

This book wouldn't have happened without so many of you. In case you don't remember who you are:

To Yousra for helping feel like my big feelings were never too much.

To Griffin for the overflowing enthusiasm you bring to all your friendships, including ours.

To Chris for being my chosen Lebanese sibling who gets those parts of me the best.

To Shae for countless massages, for so much patience, for often being my first reader, for your excellent edits despite your constant talking about not being a good editor, and for many heated games of Dutch blitz.

To Lee for the beautiful cover, for such a special friendship, and for being the person I laugh with the most.

To Wai-Yant for the beautiful studio space you've cultivated, for sharing it with me, and for multiple gossip sessions over pho.

To Helen for sending me countless articles about pain and disability when you found out what the book was going to be about (like a true dedicated Capricorn), for your constant support and excellent edits, and for countless conversations about literature and books, the fellow book nerd of my dreams.

To Ceej, for being a smart writing baby with me while we try to figure it out.

To Sasha for your supportive friendship and all the lit/book gossip and opinions.

To Hunter for being my constant companion these many years and for always calling me on my shit.

To the Gaymes group for all your love, support, attendance at readings, and the best Thursday night space of friendship I could ask for.

To Kristeen for being my biggest support and biggest fan, even when you make fun of my dad jokes.

To my mom for growing and changing with me and loving me more than I deserve.

To Tess for being such a special editor and friend, helping me get through the difficulty of trying to strive as a QPOC writer.

To Marcela for your great aesthetic eye, your sweet friendship, and our many important and nuanced money talks.

To all the folks I met during the wild Banff retreat who have become my QTBIPOC lit family.

To Ashley, my publisher, for being such a support of my work for so long, and for working so hard on this book.

This book would have never come together without the love and support of my community and for that, I'm eternally grateful.

xoxox,
Eli

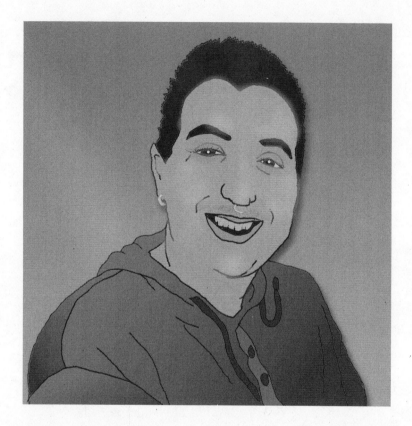

ELÌ TAREQ EL BECHELANY-LYNCH is a queer Arab poet living in Tio'tia:ke, unceded Kanien'kehá:ka territory (Montréal). Their work has appeared in *The Best Canadian Poetry* 2018 anthology, GUTS, carte blanche, the Shade Journal, The New Quarterly, Arc Poetry Magazine, Room Magazine, Cosmonauts Avenue, Plenitude, The Puritan, THEM, and Frog Hollow Press' City Series chapbook. *knot body* was shortlisted for QWF's First Book Prize in 2021. They were longlisted for the CBC poetry prize in 2019. *The Good Arabs*, their second collection, was published by Metonymy Press in 2021.